CHRONIC FATIGUE SYNDROME HANDBOOK

The Indispensable Handbook For Conquering Chronic Fatigue And Fibromyalgia, Simplified For Easy Understanding!

Vanessa Meza

Table of Contents

INTRODUCTION TO CHRONIC FATIGUE SYNDROME 2
    A. Definition Of Chronic Fatigue Syndrome (Cfs) 2
    B. Importance Of Understanding Cfs 2
    C. Overview Of The Book's Objectives 2
A. Definition of Chronic Fatigue Syndrome (CFS): 2
B. Importance of Understanding CFS: 6
C. Overview of the Book's Objectives: 8
    CHAPTER ONE 11
UNDERSTANDING CHRONIC FATIGUE SYNDROME 11
    A. History And Background Of Cfs 11
    B. Epidemiology And Prevalence 11
    C. Diagnostic Criteria And Challenges 11
    D. Current Theories And Research On The Causes Of Cfs 11
A. History and Background of CFS: 11
B. Epidemiology and Prevalence: 14
C. Diagnostic Criteria and Challenges: 16
D. Current Theories and Research on the Causes of CFS: 18
    CHAPTER TWO 21
SYMPTOMS AND IMPACT OF CHRONIC FATIGUE SYNDROME .. 21
    A. Physical Symptoms 21
    B. Cognitive Symptoms 21
    C. Emotional And Psychological Impact 21
    D. Social And Occupational Challenges 21

A. Physical Symptoms: 21

B. Cognitive Symptoms: 24

C. Emotional and Psychological Impact: 25

D. Social and Occupational Challenges: 27

CHAPTER THREE 30

DIAGNOSIS AND TREATMENT APPROACHES 30

    A. Diagnostic Process And Criteria 30

    B. Medical Tests And Examinations 30

    C. Conventional Treatment Options 30

    D. Complementary And Alternative Therapies 30

    E. Lifestyle Adjustments And Self-Care Strategies 30

A. Diagnostic Process and Criteria: 30

B. Medical Tests and Examinations: 32

C. Conventional Treatment Options: 34

D. Complementary and Alternative Therapies: 36

E. Lifestyle Adjustments and Self-Care Strategies: 37

CHAPTER FOUR 40

COPING STRATEGIES AND SUPPORT SYSTEMS 40

    A. Coping With The Limitations Of Cfs 40

    B. Building A Support Network 40

    C. Psychological Coping Techniques 40

    D. Managing Relationships And Communication 40

A. Coping with the Limitations of CFS: 40

B. Building a Support Network: 42

C. Psychological Coping Techniques: 44

D. Managing Relationships and Communication: 46

CHAPTER FIVE 49

LIVING WELL WITH CHRONIC FATIGUE SYNDROME 49

    A. Balancing Activity And Rest 49

    B. Nutrition And Exercise Considerations 49

    C. Work And Career Adjustments 49

    D. Maintaining Mental Well-Being 49

    E. Setting Realistic Goals And Expectations 49

A. Balancing Activity and Rest: 49

B. Nutrition and Exercise Considerations: 51

C. Work and Career Adjustments: 53

D. Maintaining Mental Well-Being: 55

E. Setting Realistic Goals and Expectations: 56

CHAPTER SIX 58

RESEARCH AND FUTURE DIRECTIONS 58

    A. Recent Advancements In Cfs Research 58

    B. Promising Areas Of Study 58

    C. Advocacy And Awareness Efforts 58

    D. Hope For The Future Of Cfs Treatment And Management
.... 58

A. Recent Advancements in CFS Research: 58

B. Promising Areas of Study: 61

C. Advocacy and Awareness Efforts: 64

D. Hope for the Future of CFS Treatment and Management: ... 66

PERSONAL STORIES AND PERSPECTIVES 69
    A. Narratives From Individuals Living With Cfs 69
    B. Insights From Caregivers And Loved Ones 69
    C. Success Stories And Strategies For Resilience 69
A. Narratives from Individuals Living with CFS: 69
B. Insights from Caregivers and Loved Ones: 71
C. Success Stories and Strategies for Resilience: 73
CONCLUSION 76
    A. Recap Of Key Points 76
    B. Encouragement For Readers 76
    C. Call To Action For Continued Research And Support 76
A. Recap of Key Points: 76
B. Encouragement for Readers: 78
C. Call to Action for Continued Research and Support: 79
THE END 81

INTRODUCTION TO CHRONIC FATIGUE SYNDROME

A. Definition Of Chronic Fatigue Syndrome (Cfs)

B. Importance Of Understanding Cfs

C. Overview Of The Book's Objectives

A. Definition of Chronic Fatigue Syndrome (CFS):

Chronic Fatigue Syndrome (CFS), also known as Myalgic Encephalomyelitis (ME), is a complex and debilitating disorder characterized primarily by extreme fatigue or tiredness that doesn't improve with rest and may worsen with physical or mental activity. The fatigue experienced by individuals with CFS is often severe enough to interfere with their daily activities and can't be explained by any underlying medical condition.

Alongside persistent fatigue, CFS is typically associated with a range of other symptoms, including but not limited to:

Post-exertional malaise (PEM): Worsening of symptoms after physical or mental exertion.

Unrefreshing sleep: Despite spending long hours in bed, individuals with CFS often wake up feeling unrefreshed and fatigued.

Cognitive difficulties: Often referred to as "brain fog," individuals may experience problems with memory, concentration, and word retrieval.

Muscle and joint pain: Persistent pain in muscles and joints without any apparent cause.

Headaches: Frequent and severe headaches are common in CFS patients.

Sore throat and swollen lymph nodes: Some individuals may experience these symptoms as well.

It's important to note that there's no specific test to diagnose CFS. Diagnosis is typically made by excluding other potential causes of fatigue and assessing symptoms based on established criteria, such as the Fukuda criteria or the more recent International Consensus Criteria (ICC) for ME.

B. Importance of Understanding CFS:

Understanding Chronic Fatigue Syndrome is crucial for several reasons:

Quality of Life: CFS can severely impact an individual's quality of life, making it difficult to perform daily tasks, work, or engage in social activities.

Misdiagnosis: Without proper understanding, CFS may be misdiagnosed as depression or other medical conditions, leading to inappropriate treatment and prolonged suffering.

Research and Treatment: Improved understanding of CFS is essential for advancing research into its causes, mechanisms, and potential treatments. Currently, there's no cure for CFS, and treatment focuses on managing symptoms and improving quality of life.

Public Awareness: Increasing awareness about CFS helps reduce stigma surrounding the condition and promotes empathy and support for individuals living with it.

Healthcare Resource Allocation: Understanding the prevalence and impact of CFS helps allocate healthcare resources more effectively to support affected individuals.

C. Overview of the Book's Objectives:

The objectives of a book on Chronic Fatigue Syndrome may vary depending on its focus and audience. However, common objectives might include:

Educating Readers: Providing comprehensive information about CFS, including its symptoms, diagnosis, treatment options, and coping strategies.

Raising Awareness: Increasing public and healthcare professional awareness about the realities of living with CFS and the challenges faced by individuals with the condition.

Promoting Empathy: Encouraging empathy and understanding towards individuals with CFS, their caregivers, and support networks.

Offering Practical Guidance: Offering practical advice and tools for managing CFS symptoms, navigating healthcare systems, and accessing support services.

Highlighting Research: Summarizing current research findings on CFS, including potential causes, risk factors, and emerging treatments.

Advocating for Change: Advocating for improved healthcare policies, increased funding for CFS research, and better support services for affected individuals.

CHAPTER ONE

UNDERSTANDING CHRONIC FATIGUE SYNDROME

A. History And Background Of Cfs

B. Epidemiology And Prevalence

C. Diagnostic Criteria And Challenges

D. Current Theories And Research On The Causes Of Cfs

A. History and Background of CFS:

Chronic Fatigue Syndrome (CFS) has a complex history marked by changing names, diagnostic criteria, and understanding. Here's a brief overview:

Early Observations: Reports of a mysterious illness resembling CFS date back to the early 20th century, but it gained significant attention in the 1980s and 1990s.

Various Names: CFS has been known by various names, including myalgic encephalomyelitis (ME), post-viral fatigue syndrome, and systemic exertion intolerance disease (SEID).

1988 CDC Definition: The Centers for Disease Control and Prevention (CDC) provided the first formal definition of CFS in 1988, emphasizing the importance of fatigue lasting for at least six months and the exclusion of other medical or psychiatric conditions.

Controversies and Stigma: CFS has faced controversies and skepticism, with some medical professionals questioning its legitimacy as a distinct illness. Stigma surrounding the condition has also affected patients' experiences and access to care.

Advances in Understanding: Over the years, advances in research have led to a better understanding of CFS as a complex multi-system disorder involving dysregulation of the immune, endocrine, and neurological systems.

B. Epidemiology and Prevalence:

Determining the exact prevalence of CFS is challenging due to variations in diagnostic criteria, underreporting, and misdiagnosis. However, studies suggest the following:

Prevalence: Estimates of CFS prevalence vary widely, ranging from 0.1% to 2.5% of the population, depending on the criteria used and the population studied.

Demographic Factors: CFS affects people of all ages, races, and socioeconomic backgrounds, but it's more common in women than men. The onset often occurs in early to mid-adulthood, but it can affect children and adolescents as well.

Impact on Daily Life: CFS can have a profound impact on individuals' daily lives, impairing their ability to work, attend school, engage in social activities, and maintain relationships.

C. Diagnostic Criteria and Challenges:

Diagnosing CFS remains challenging due to the absence of specific diagnostic tests and the overlap of symptoms with other medical conditions. Some key diagnostic criteria and challenges include:

Fukuda Criteria: The Fukuda criteria, established in 1994, are widely used for diagnosing CFS. They require the presence of severe, unexplained fatigue lasting for at least six months, along with specific accompanying symptoms.

International Consensus Criteria (ICC): More recent criteria, such as the ICC, emphasize post-exertional malaise (PEM) and neurocognitive symptoms as hallmark features of CFS.

Overlap with Other Conditions: CFS shares symptoms with several other medical conditions, including fibromyalgia, autoimmune disorders, and mood disorders, leading to misdiagnosis and delayed diagnosis.

Diagnostic Delays: Many individuals with CFS experience significant delays in diagnosis, often enduring years of uncertainty and frustration before receiving a proper diagnosis.

D. Current Theories and Research on the Causes of CFS:

Despite decades of research, the exact causes of CFS remain elusive. However, several theories and areas of research have emerged, including:

Viral Infections: Some researchers speculate that viral infections, such as Epstein-Barr virus (EBV) or human herpesvirus 6 (HHV-6), may trigger or contribute to the development of CFS in susceptible individuals.

Immune Dysfunction: Dysregulation of the immune system, including chronic inflammation and abnormalities in cytokine levels, has been observed in individuals with CFS, suggesting an immune component to the illness.

Neuroendocrine Abnormalities: Abnormalities in the hypothalamic-pituitary-adrenal (HPA) axis and other neuroendocrine systems have been documented in CFS patients, indicating disruptions in stress response and hormone regulation.

Genetic Predisposition: There may be a genetic predisposition to CFS, as evidenced by familial clustering and genetic studies identifying potential susceptibility genes.

Dysautonomia: Some researchers propose that dysautonomia, dysfunction of the autonomic nervous system, may play a role in the development of CFS symptoms, such as orthostatic intolerance and cardiovascular abnormalities.

CHAPTER TWO

SYMPTOMS AND IMPACT OF CHRONIC FATIGUE SYNDROME

A. Physical Symptoms

B. Cognitive Symptoms

C. Emotional And Psychological Impact

D. Social And Occupational Challenges

A. Physical Symptoms: Chronic Fatigue Syndrome (CFS) is characterized by a wide range of physical symptoms that can vary in severity and duration. Some common physical symptoms include:

Persistent Fatigue: Overwhelming fatigue that is not relieved by rest and significantly impairs daily functioning.

Post-exertional Malaise (PEM): Worsening of symptoms after physical or mental exertion, often lasting for days or weeks.

Muscle and Joint Pain: Persistent pain and soreness in muscles and joints, without evidence of inflammation or injury.

Headaches: Frequent and severe headaches, including migraines, are common in individuals with CFS.

Unrefreshing Sleep: Despite spending long hours in bed, CFS patients often wake up feeling unrefreshed and fatigued.

Dizziness and Orthostatic Intolerance: Symptoms such as dizziness, lightheadedness, and fainting upon standing up, indicating dysfunction in the autonomic nervous system.

Gastrointestinal Disturbances: Some individuals with CFS may experience symptoms such as nausea, bloating, diarrhea, or constipation.

B. Cognitive Symptoms:

CFS can also affect cognitive functioning, leading to difficulties with concentration, memory, and information processing. Common cognitive symptoms include:

Brain Fog:

A subjective feeling of mental cloudiness or confusion, making it challenging to think clearly or concentrate on tasks.

Memory Problems: Difficulty remembering things, including recent events, names, or information previously known.

Word Retrieval Issues: Difficulty finding the right words or expressing thoughts verbally, sometimes referred to as "tip-of-the-tongue" phenomenon.

Slowed Processing Speed: Cognitive tasks may take longer to complete, and individuals may feel mentally sluggish or "stuck" when trying to problem-solve or make decisions.

C. Emotional and Psychological Impact:

Living with CFS can take a significant toll on one's emotional and psychological well-being. Some emotional and psychological effects include:

Depression and Anxiety: Chronic fatigue and physical limitations can lead to feelings of sadness, hopelessness, and anxiety about the future.

Social Withdrawal: Difficulty participating in social activities due to fatigue and other symptoms may lead to isolation and feelings of loneliness.

Frustration and Loss of Independence: Struggling with symptoms and limitations can be frustrating and may result in a loss of independence and autonomy.

Stress and Coping Challenges: Managing the demands of daily life while dealing with CFS can be stressful, and finding effective coping strategies may be challenging.

D. Social and Occupational Challenges:

CFS can profoundly impact an individual's social relationships and ability to work or pursue educational goals. Some social and occupational challenges include:

Work Limitations: Many individuals with CFS are unable to work or have reduced work hours due to fatigue and other symptoms, leading to financial strain and career disruptions.

Educational Challenges: CFS may interfere with academic performance and attendance, affecting educational goals and future opportunities.

Strained Relationships: Managing relationships with family, friends, and partners can be challenging when dealing with the unpredictable nature of CFS symptoms and limitations.

Stigmatization and Misunderstanding: CFS is often poorly understood by others, leading to stigmatization, skepticism, and invalidation of the individual's experiences.

CHAPTER THREE

DIAGNOSIS AND TREATMENT APPROACHES

A. Diagnostic Process And Criteria

B. Medical Tests And Examinations

C. Conventional Treatment Options

D. Complementary And Alternative Therapies

E. Lifestyle Adjustments And Self-Care Strategies

A. Diagnostic Process and Criteria:

Diagnosing CFS can be challenging due to the absence of specific diagnostic tests and the overlap of symptoms with other medical conditions. The diagnostic process typically involves the following steps:

Medical History and Physical Examination: Healthcare providers will take a detailed medical history and perform a physical examination to rule out other medical conditions that could be causing the symptoms.

Diagnostic Criteria: Diagnosis of CFS is based on established criteria, such as the Fukuda criteria or the International Consensus Criteria (ICC), which require the presence of persistent fatigue and specific accompanying symptoms for a certain duration.

Exclusion of Other Conditions: CFS is a diagnosis of exclusion, meaning other medical or psychiatric conditions that could explain the symptoms must be ruled out through appropriate testing and evaluation.

B. Medical Tests and Examinations:

While there is no specific laboratory test for diagnosing CFS, healthcare providers may order various tests to rule out other potential causes of fatigue and related symptoms. These tests may include:

Blood Tests: To check for infections, autoimmune disorders, thyroid dysfunction, and other medical conditions.

Imaging Studies: Such as MRI or CT scans, to evaluate the brain and other organs for abnormalities.

Sleep Studies: To assess for sleep disorders that could contribute to fatigue and unrefreshing sleep.

Cardiopulmonary Testing: To evaluate heart and lung function, particularly in individuals experiencing symptoms such as dizziness or shortness of breath.

C. Conventional Treatment Options:

Treatment for CFS focuses on managing symptoms and improving quality of life. Conventional treatment options may include:

Medications: Such as pain relievers for muscle and joint pain, sleep aids for insomnia, and antidepressants or antianxiety medications for mood disturbances.

Cognitive Behavioral Therapy (CBT): A type of psychotherapy that helps individuals cope with CFS symptoms and improve their functioning through changes in thoughts, behaviors, and emotions.

Graded Exercise Therapy (GET): A structured exercise program designed to gradually increase physical activity levels while avoiding overexertion, with the goal of improving stamina and reducing symptoms.

Occupational Therapy: To help individuals adapt their daily activities and routines to manage fatigue and conserve energy.

D. Complementary and Alternative Therapies:

Some individuals with CFS may explore complementary and alternative therapies to complement conventional treatment approaches. These may include:

Acupuncture: Some people find relief from symptoms such as pain and fatigue through acupuncture, a traditional Chinese medicine practice involving the insertion of thin needles into specific points on the body.

Massage Therapy: Massage therapy can help reduce muscle tension, alleviate pain, and promote relaxation.

Nutritional Supplements: Certain supplements, such as magnesium, vitamin D, and coenzyme Q10, are sometimes used to support energy production and overall health in individuals with CFS. However, evidence for their effectiveness is limited.

E. Lifestyle Adjustments and Self-Care Strategies:

Lifestyle adjustments and self-care strategies play a crucial role in managing CFS symptoms and improving overall well-being. These may include:

Pacing: Learning to balance activity and rest to avoid overexertion and PEM.

Stress Management: Techniques such as mindfulness, meditation, and relaxation exercises can help reduce stress and promote relaxation.

Sleep Hygiene: Establishing healthy sleep habits and routines to improve the quality of sleep and reduce fatigue.

Nutrition: Eating a balanced diet rich in fruits, vegetables, whole grains, and lean proteins to support overall health and energy levels.

Supportive Relationships: Seeking support from family, friends, support groups, and mental health professionals can provide emotional support and practical assistance in coping with CFS.

CHAPTER FOUR

COPING STRATEGIES AND SUPPORT SYSTEMS

A. Coping With The Limitations Of Cfs

B. Building A Support Network

C. Psychological Coping Techniques

D. Managing Relationships And Communication

A. Coping with the Limitations of CFS:

Coping with the limitations imposed by CFS can be challenging, but there are several strategies that individuals can employ:

Acceptance: Acknowledge the reality of living with CFS and accept that certain limitations may be present. Acceptance doesn't mean resignation but rather recognizing what is within one's control and finding ways to adapt.

Pacing: Learn to pace activities and prioritize tasks to avoid overexertion and minimize symptoms of fatigue and post-exertional malaise (PEM). Break tasks into smaller, manageable chunks and take frequent breaks as needed.

Adaptation: Modify daily routines, work schedules, and social activities to accommodate the fluctuating nature of CFS symptoms. Be flexible and willing to adjust plans as needed.

Self-compassion: Be kind to yourself and practice self-compassion. Recognize that living with CFS can be challenging, and it's okay to ask for help and take breaks when needed.

B. Building a Support Network: Building a strong support network can provide invaluable emotional, practical, and social support for individuals living with CFS. Here are some ways to build and maintain a support network:

Family and Friends: Lean on supportive family members and friends who understand and empathize with your experience. Communicate openly with them about your needs and limitations.

Support Groups: Joining a support group for individuals with CFS can provide a sense of belonging, validation, and shared understanding. Connect with others who are facing similar challenges and share experiences, tips, and resources.

Online Communities: Participate in online forums, social media groups, and virtual support networks dedicated to CFS. Engage with others, ask questions, and offer support to fellow members.

Healthcare Providers: Build a collaborative relationship with healthcare providers who are knowledgeable about CFS and can offer guidance, treatment, and support.

C. Psychological Coping Techniques:

Psychological coping techniques can help individuals manage stress, anxiety, and other emotional challenges associated with CFS. Some effective techniques include:

Mindfulness and Meditation: Practice mindfulness meditation, deep breathing exercises, or progressive muscle relaxation to promote relaxation, reduce stress, and increase self-awareness.

Cognitive Restructuring: Challenge negative thoughts and beliefs about CFS by reframing them in a more balanced and realistic way. Focus on cultivating a positive and hopeful mindset.

Journaling: Keep a journal to express thoughts, feelings, and experiences related to living with CFS. Writing can be a therapeutic outlet for processing emotions and gaining insights into coping strategies.

Creative Expression: Engage in creative activities such as art, music, or writing as a means of self-expression and emotional release.

D. Managing Relationships and Communication:

Maintaining healthy relationships and effective communication can be crucial for navigating the challenges of living with CFS. Here are some tips for managing relationships:

Open Communication: Communicate openly and honestly with loved ones about your experiences, limitations, and needs related to CFS. Encourage dialogue and mutual understanding.

Setting Boundaries: Set boundaries with family, friends, and coworkers regarding your energy levels, activity limitations, and need for rest. Be assertive in advocating for your needs and priorities.

Educating Others: Educate family members, friends, and colleagues about CFS to increase awareness and understanding. Provide them with information about the condition, its symptoms, and how they can offer support.

Seeking Professional Help: Consider seeking couples counseling or family therapy to address relationship challenges related to CFS. A qualified therapist can help facilitate communication, problem-solving, and conflict resolution.

CHAPTER FIVE

LIVING WELL WITH CHRONIC FATIGUE SYNDROME

A. Balancing Activity And Rest

B. Nutrition And Exercise Considerations

C. Work And Career Adjustments

D. Maintaining Mental Well-Being

E. Setting Realistic Goals And Expectations

A. Balancing Activity and Rest: Balancing activity and rest is essential for managing CFS symptoms and conserving energy. Here are some strategies:

Pacing: Break tasks into smaller, manageable chunks, and alternate periods of activity with periods of rest to avoid overexertion.

Listen to Your Body: Pay attention to your body's signals and adjust your activity levels accordingly. Rest when you need to, and don't push yourself beyond your limits.

Schedule Rest Breaks: Incorporate regular rest breaks throughout the day, especially during periods of increased activity or when experiencing symptoms of fatigue.

Prioritize Activities: Identify the most important tasks and activities and prioritize them, focusing on what needs to be done rather than what you would like to do.

B. Nutrition and Exercise Considerations:

Proper nutrition and gentle exercise can support overall health and well-being for individuals with CFS:

Healthy Eating: Follow a balanced diet rich in fruits, vegetables, whole grains, lean proteins, and healthy fats to provide essential nutrients and support energy levels.

Hydration: Drink plenty of water throughout the day to stay hydrated and help combat fatigue.

Gentle Exercise: Engage in gentle forms of exercise such as walking, yoga, tai chi, or swimming, tailored to your individual abilities and tolerance levels. Start slowly and gradually increase intensity as tolerated.

Avoid Overexertion: Be mindful not to overexert yourself during exercise or physical activity. Listen to your body and stop if you experience excessive fatigue or worsening symptoms.

C. Work and Career Adjustments: Managing work and career responsibilities with CFS may require adjustments and accommodations:

Flexible Work Arrangements: Explore options for flexible work schedules, remote work, part-time hours, or job sharing to accommodate fluctuations in energy levels and symptoms.

Open Communication: Communicate openly with your employer or supervisor about your condition and any accommodations you may need. Discuss strategies for managing workload and responsibilities effectively.

Pacing at Work: Pace yourself at work by prioritizing tasks, taking regular breaks, and incorporating rest periods into your schedule as needed.

Seek Support: Seek support from your employer's human resources department, occupational health services, or disability accommodations office to explore available resources and support options.

D. Maintaining Mental Well-Being:

Taking care of your mental well-being is essential for coping with the challenges of living with CFS:

Stress Management: Practice stress-reduction techniques such as mindfulness, meditation, deep breathing exercises, or progressive muscle relaxation to promote relaxation and reduce anxiety.

Self-Care: Prioritize self-care activities that promote relaxation and enjoyment, such as hobbies, spending time with loved ones, or engaging in activities that bring you joy.

Professional Support: Consider seeking support from a therapist or counselor who specializes in chronic illness or pain management. Therapy can provide a safe space to explore emotions, develop coping strategies, and receive validation and support.

E. Setting Realistic Goals and Expectations:

Setting realistic goals and expectations is important for managing CFS and preventing frustration and disappointment:

Set Priorities: Identify your most important goals and focus your energy on pursuing those that align with your values and priorities.

Be Flexible: Be willing to adjust your goals and expectations in response to changes in your health, energy levels, and symptoms.

Celebrate Progress: Acknowledge and celebrate small victories and accomplishments along the way, even if they may seem minor. Recognize your resilience and perseverance in the face of challenges.

CHAPTER SIX

RESEARCH AND FUTURE DIRECTIONS

A. Recent Advancements In Cfs Research

B. Promising Areas Of Study

C. Advocacy And Awareness Efforts

D. Hope For The Future Of Cfs Treatment And Management

A. Recent Advancements in CFS Research:

In recent years, there have been several notable advancements in CFS research, including:

Biological Markers: Researchers have identified potential biological markers associated with CFS, such as abnormalities in immune function, inflammation, gene expression, and metabolic pathways. These markers may help improve diagnosis, subtyping, and treatment approaches.

Neuroimaging Studies: Advances in neuroimaging techniques, such as functional MRI (fMRI) and positron emission tomography (PET), have provided insights into brain abnormalities and dysfunctions associated with CFS, including altered brain structure, connectivity, and function.

Microbiome Research: Studies investigating the gut microbiome in individuals with CFS have revealed alterations in microbial composition and diversity, suggesting a potential link between gut health and CFS symptoms. Further research in this area may lead to novel therapeutic interventions.

Immunotherapy Trials: Clinical trials investigating immunomodulatory therapies, such as monoclonal antibodies and immune checkpoint inhibitors, have shown promising results in some individuals with CFS, highlighting the potential role of immune dysregulation in the pathogenesis of the condition.

B. Promising Areas of Study:
Several promising areas of study are currently being explored in CFS research, including:

Precision Medicine: Advancements in genomics, proteomics, and metabolomics are paving the way for personalized medicine approaches in CFS, allowing for targeted interventions based on individual molecular profiles and disease subtypes.

Neuroinflammation: Increasing evidence suggests that neuroinflammation may play a key role in the pathophysiology of CFS. Targeting neuroinflammatory pathways and neuroimmune interactions may offer new avenues for treatment development.

Mitochondrial Dysfunction: Dysfunction of mitochondrial energy metabolism has been implicated in CFS. Research focusing on mitochondrial function and bioenergetics may uncover novel therapeutic targets for improving energy production and reducing fatigue.

Psychoneuroimmunology: Investigating the complex interactions between the immune system, nervous system, and psychological factors in CFS may provide insights into the underlying mechanisms and inform multidisciplinary treatment approaches.

C. Advocacy and Awareness Efforts:

Advocacy organizations and patient advocacy groups play a crucial role in raising awareness, promoting research, and advocating for the needs of individuals with CFS. Efforts to increase advocacy and awareness include:

Educational Campaigns: Organizations such as the Solve ME/CFS Initiative, MEAction, and #MEAction Network work to raise public awareness about CFS, educate healthcare providers, and advocate for increased research funding and support.

Patient Advocacy: CFS patients and advocates share their stories, participate in research initiatives, and advocate for improved healthcare policies and access to care for individuals with CFS.

Community Engagement: Building a supportive community of patients, caregivers, researchers, and healthcare professionals fosters collaboration, sharing of resources, and mutual support in the fight against CFS.

D. Hope for the Future of CFS Treatment and Management:

Despite the challenges, there is reason for hope in the future of CFS treatment and management:

Advancing Research: Ongoing research efforts continue to uncover new insights into the underlying mechanisms of CFS and identify potential therapeutic targets. Collaborative research initiatives, such as the National Institutes of Health (NIH) Intramural Study on ME/CFS and the UK ME/CFS Biobank, are driving progress in the field.

Patient-Centered Care:

A growing recognition of the importance of patient-centered care and shared decision-making is leading to more holistic and individualized approaches to managing CFS. Empowering patients to play an active role in their healthcare and treatment decisions is key to improving outcomes.

Emerging Therapies: Promising therapies, including immunomodulatory agents, mitochondrial-targeted treatments, and interventions targeting neuroinflammatory pathways, are being explored in clinical trials. While further research is needed to confirm efficacy and safety, these therapies offer hope for future treatment options.

PERSONAL STORIES AND PERSPECTIVES

A. Narratives From Individuals Living With Cfs

B. Insights From Caregivers And Loved Ones

C. Success Stories And Strategies For Resilience

A. Narratives from Individuals Living with CFS:

Sharing personal narratives and lived experiences can help raise awareness, foster understanding, and provide support for individuals living with CFS. Some common themes in these narratives include:

Struggles with Diagnosis: Many individuals with CFS recount the challenges they faced in obtaining a diagnosis, including skepticism from healthcare providers, misdiagnosis, and delays in receiving appropriate care.

Impact on Daily Life: Personal stories often highlight the profound impact of CFS on various aspects of daily life, including work, relationships, social activities, and mental well-being.

Coping Strategies: Individuals share their strategies for coping with symptoms, managing limitations, and finding moments of joy and fulfillment despite the challenges of living with CFS.

Advocacy and Empowerment: Many individuals with CFS become advocates for themselves and others, sharing their stories, participating in research initiatives, and advocating for increased awareness, support, and research funding.

B. Insights from Caregivers and Loved Ones:

Caregivers and loved ones play a crucial role in supporting individuals with CFS and navigating the challenges of the condition. Insights from caregivers and loved ones may include:

Support and Understanding: Caregivers share their experiences of providing emotional, practical, and social support to their loved ones with CFS, including the importance of empathy, patience, and active listening.

Challenges and Adjustments: Caregivers discuss the challenges they face in balancing their own needs and responsibilities with those of their loved ones with CFS, as well as the adjustments they make to accommodate the fluctuating nature of the condition.

Advocacy and Awareness: Caregivers often become advocates for individuals with CFS, raising awareness, educating others, and advocating for improved healthcare services, research funding, and support networks.

C. Success Stories and Strategies for Resilience:

Despite the challenges of living with CFS, many individuals share success stories and strategies for resilience that offer hope and inspiration. These may include:

Finding Meaning and Purpose: Individuals with CFS share how they have found meaning and purpose in their lives despite the limitations imposed by the condition, whether through creative pursuits, advocacy work, or supporting others.

Building Support Networks: Success stories often highlight the importance of building supportive relationships, connecting with others who understand and empathize with their experiences, and accessing peer support groups and online communities.

Embracing Self-Care: Individuals discuss the importance of self-care practices such as pacing, mindfulness, nutrition, and gentle exercise in managing symptoms, improving well-being, and fostering resilience.

Celebrating Achievements: Success stories celebrate achievements, no matter how small, and acknowledge the strength, courage, and resilience of individuals living with CFS in the face of adversity.

CONCLUSION

A. Recap Of Key Points

B. Encouragement For Readers

C. Call To Action For Continued Research And Support

A. Recap of Key Points:

Throughout this exploration of Chronic Fatigue Syndrome (CFS), we've covered various aspects of the condition, including its definition, symptoms, diagnosis, treatment, coping strategies, and future directions. Key points include:

CFS is a complex and debilitating condition characterized by persistent fatigue and a range of physical, cognitive, and emotional symptoms.

Diagnosis of CFS requires careful evaluation and exclusion of other medical conditions, often leading to challenges and delays in diagnosis.

Treatment approaches focus on symptom management, lifestyle adjustments, and holistic care to improve quality of life for individuals with CFS.

Coping strategies, support networks, and advocacy efforts play crucial roles in helping individuals living with CFS navigate the challenges of the condition and foster resilience.

B. Encouragement for Readers:
To individuals living with CFS and their loved ones, it's essential to remember that you are not alone in your journey. While living with CFS can be incredibly challenging, there is hope, support, and resources available to help you navigate the ups and downs. Embrace self-compassion, prioritize self-care, and celebrate your strengths and achievements, no matter how small. Together, we can raise awareness, promote understanding, and advocate

for improved care and support for individuals affected by CFS.

C. Call to Action for Continued Research and Support:

As we conclude, let us not forget the importance of continued research, advocacy, and support for individuals with CFS. Researchers, healthcare providers, policymakers, and advocacy organizations must work together to advance our understanding of the underlying mechanisms of CFS, improve diagnosis and treatment options, and address the unmet needs of individuals living with the condition.

By raising awareness, supporting research initiatives, and advocating for increased funding and resources, we can make a difference in the lives of those affected by CFS and move closer toward a future where effective treatments and support systems are available for all.

THE END

www.ingramcontent.com/pod-product-compliance
Lightning Source LLC
Chambersburg PA
CBHW070313230526
45470CB00002B/851